Testimonials

I love your book! I learned so much in a fun way. There are things I never would have thought about and some tips that will help me going forward.

—S.H.

Your book is amazing! I know it will be a beautiful resource for other Caregivers.

—D.H.

Thank you so much for your Packing List. You have things on there that I have not thought of.

—M.T.

I love your book! It is even more complete than I thought possible—you thought of everything.

—L.M.

Amy, as you lovingly take care of others, remember to take care of yourself.

Barb

The
Caregiver's
Guidebook

Your Resource for Successfully Navigating Life as a Caregiver

BARBARA A. STEWART

IMB Press

The Caregiver's Guidebook
Your Resource for Successfully Navigating Life as a Caregiver
By Barbara A. Stewart
IMB Press

Published by IMB Press, Cary, Illinois

Cover and Interior design: Davis Creative, www.DavisCreative.com

Publisher's Cataloging-In-Publication Data

(Prepared by The Donohue Group, Inc.)

Names: Stewart, Barbara A., 1954- author.
Title: The caregiver's guidebook : your resource for successfully navigating life as a caregiver / Barbara A. Stewart.
Description: Cary, Illinois : IMB Press, [2019]
Identifiers: ISBN 9781733903103 (paperback) | ISBN 9781733903110 (ebook)
Subjects: LCSH: Caregivers--Psychology--Handbooks, manuals, etc. | Caregivers--Health and hygiene--Handbooks, manuals, etc. | BISAC: HEALTH & FITNESS / Health Care Issues. | MEDICAL / Caregiving. | BODY, MIND & SPIRIT / Inspiration & Personal Growth.
Classification: LCC RA645.3 .S74 2019 (print) | LCC RA645.3 (ebook) | DDC 649.8--dc23

This book is dedicated to Caregivers for sharing their personal stories, and for helping me understand the depth of being a Caregiver through examples of compassion, strength, and endurance.

TABLE OF CONTENTS

Introduction

If your new journey creates frustration, concern, or a quest for guidance on *how to do it right*, know that you are not alone. In fact, you are the reason for this book! When I became a Caregiver, I felt like I was embarking on a journey with no road map. Most Caregivers blindly trudge through whatever comes their way and most often do an incredible job with no expectations of reward or recognition. I often hear Caregivers label themselves as *just* a Caregiver. It is probably why we do not share our experiences about the simple tasks that are associated with the care and nurturing of our loved ones.

The purpose of *The Caregiver's Guidebook* is not to solely provide you with my story, but to share worksheets that will enable you to chronicle, organize, and personalize your own story. I want to share our similarities and honor our differences. I want you to understand the healthcare system and how to navigate both physically and emotionally. I want you to be able to be organized as you nurture the well being of your loved one *and* yourself. I want you to have a voice and not feel so alone. I want you to have confidence, concern for self-care, and hope for better days ahead.

My Story

Most of us have been surrounded by Caregivers throughout our lives, yet we have not given much thought to this complex role or the tasks related to this unsolicited title.

In 2013, I suddenly and unexpectedly began my own journey as a Caregiver when my husband was diagnosed with end-stage liver failure. It was then that reality hit me like a ton of bricks, as my life was about to change dramatically. I did not want to be called a Caregiver since I did not know what it meant, let alone how to be one! The choice, however, was not mine to make.

I interviewed other Caregivers with full intent that they would provide me with instructions, and perhaps a magical book that would have all the answers to my questions. I did receive valuable information about medical processes, and the roller coaster of new feelings and tasks that become the new normal. I now know this role to be an obvious dedication of love, concern, and compassion that keeps the Caregiver going on a selfless path with purpose. There were numerous similarities among these Caregivers, yet more often, a uniqueness of family dynamics, patient's response, and type of illness or injury.

My most vivid memory throughout these interviews, sparked by the newness of this role and perhaps my naivety was—I just wanted to know where to park. I kept thinking that perhaps I was focusing on the small things that obviously had simple answers. I found this to be quite the opposite and became grateful for my curiosity and assertiveness in my search to make some sense out of this chaotic simplicity.

Throughout my time at a big hospital in a big city and away from the comforts of home, I realized that I felt quite unequipped. Again, naively, I often thought it odd that simple inquiries like, "where can I send a fax", or, "where can I park", seemed daunting. I felt certain that I could not be the first person who needed this information and that I would find answers—eventually. I suppose the advantage of a lengthy stay allowed me to begin my quest of collecting key information to make my days and weeks at the hospital easier and more efficient. To this day, I continue to have conversations with other Caregivers about the confusion and frustration of logistics and navigation.

This process and all the experiences moving forward led me to the creation of this Caregiver's guidebook. My intent is to provide all Caregivers with references, guidance, comfort, and most of all a voice, from diagnosis through follow up. With all due respect to the advancement and intricacies of the medical world, I can only hope that Caregivers can continue to be recognized as an integrated part of the health care process.

After several years of tests and procedures, advancements, and setbacks, my husband had a liver transplant in 2016. Almost three years later, he is doing well. Both of our lives have changed and will be different from this experience. I am lucky that my husband was positive throughout his journey, and that the intensity of my caregiving experience was a relatively short jaunt. My heart goes out to those Caregivers whose journey becomes long term. I now know that I will always have the title of Caregiver. I have learned a lot about caregiving, and that it is not so bad once you learn the ropes. I have learned about life, and I have learned about people and processes. I realize that we all have a story—which is the real magic that connects us.

May you always find a place to park

Concerned
Attentive
Reliable
Efficient
Grateful
Intuitive
Visible
Engaged
Responsible

What is a Caregiver

Everyone seems to have heard the word Caregiver, but we seem to struggle with being able to define it. Typically, there is not a place to go to learn how to be one. Each situation has similarities to one another; however, your story can have components that are like no other.

Official definitions of a Caregiver sound simple:

A Caregiver is a family member or paid helper who regularly looks after and gives assistance to someone that is sick, elderly or disabled.

A Caregiver is someone that nurtures your well-being physically, mentally, socially, or financially, on a professional or personal level.

At times you are presented with the role of a Caregiver on a random day (car accident, heart attack, organ failure). This instantly becomes your new life.

Sometimes you are eased into the role of a Caregiver with hints of a situation that forms over time (Alzheimer's, elder care, special needs).

For some, being a Caregiver is not a title or label they would bestow upon themselves. Rather it is an expectation, a tradition, or simply just *something you do*. Whether you are a parent who takes care of your family, an adult child who holds a hand, sings a song or reads a story, or you perform a simple neighborly deed...*it is still considered caregiving*.

Regardless of how you become blessed with this new title, what your dynamics are, or how much you learn through others, we all share a common denominator:

Your Health and Well Being Are Affected

If the family were a fruit,
it would be an orange,
a circle of sections held together
but separable—
each segment distinct.

Letty Cottin-Pogrebin

Caregiving Dynamics

There will be many changes in your life as you now know it. The impact of these changes depends on components that are already in place, or the things that you have never thought about.

In most cases you and your loved one are presented with an illness or injury that you are not familiar with, and in some cases have never heard of. Try to embrace this as part of your new journey as you learn all about this diagnosis and how it affects the rest of the body, as well as what is needed to heal. Try to reach out with more than just computer research, such as, connecting with groups or individuals that have experienced similar adversities, or by visiting medical libraries which are often located in some of the major big city hospitals.

The following list of questions will help you determine if you are "ready" to become a Caregiver and understand what you are ready for. This list also contains some of the top concerns of a Caregiver, although most of us only become aware of them as they occur. Do not feel as though you need to answer all these questions at once. This list is meant to guide you step by step through your new journey. Having an awareness and keeping this list handy will most certainly ease the shock, uncertainty, unpreparedness, and possibility of overlooking key areas when the need arises. You will have a much better chance of embracing the "new you".

CAREGIVING DYNAMICS:

Questions to Consider

- What is your relationship to the patient?
- Will you be the main caregiver?
- Do you live with the patient?
- Do you live nearby?
- Are you organized?
- Are you assertive?
- Do you already take good care of yourself?
- What is your financial status?
- Do you know the financial status of the patient?
- Will you be the only one taking care of this person?
- What does your normal day look like?
- Will you be responsible for taking this person to appointments?
- Does the patient have organized and accessible records?
- Has the patient talked with you about their care?
- Do all family members understand and agree with the Plan?
- Have you been in the medical setting before?
- Do you have access to insurance policies (medical & prescription)?

- Do you have power of attorney? (medical and financial)
- Are you set up for impromptu hospital stays?
- Do you need referrals?
- Can you take pictures with your phone?
- Are you going to be able to shop and cook for special meals?
- Do you have good nutrition in place for yourself?
- Do you have a reliable vehicle?
- Do you know how to ask for help?
- Do you know what to ask help for?
- Is the home where the patient is staying clean and safe?
- Are you okay with travel in bad weather?
- Do you have a list of what to bring on hospital stays both planned and impromptu?
- Do you know who to call after hours?
- Do you have contacts set up in your phone (numbers & email)?
- Do you have someone set up to take care of pets, mail, lights?
- Is your place of employment aware of your new lifestyle?
- Do you have a network established: family, friends, health care?

- Do you have someone in place to be the Caregiver if you are sick?
- Do you have an action plan for the next phase?
- Do you have an action plan for the unexpected?
- Did you consider a life alert device and/or medical bracelet?
- Do you have a list of current medications posted in several locations?
- Do you have a notification site set up to disseminate the patient's health status?
- Do you have a familiarity with this illness or injury?
- Are you aware of forms that your hospital requires to enable you to make and discuss health decisions for the patient?
- Are you comfortable discussing health changes with the patient?
- Do you have a way to efficiently communicate with others?
- Do you know who to talk to if you cannot answer these questions?
- Do you have a Plan B?

To protect your energy
It's okay to...
cancel a commitment,
not answer a call,
change your mind,
want to be alone,
take a day off,
do nothing,
speak up,
let go.

How Caregiving Affects You

Several things start to happen in your new role as a Caregiver. Some of these things happen right away, some of them over time, some you notice, and some take over like a sleeping demon that appears in full force right when you are at your weakest point. Once again, awareness is the key to maintaining an even keel, or at least as close to it as you can. Awareness is also the component that enables you to ask for help as you notice yourself losing control over your new normal.

My conversations with new Caregivers sparked feelings in me that resonated quite profoundly. "I do not know what to do next" or "I'm overwhelmed" are desperate, emotional, yet quite common statements from Caregivers at the onset of their new journey. Everything I had to do seemed to be of equal importance and urgency. A professional that I reached out to, suggested that I focus on only one, two, or three things on my list, then begin to reach out to others for help in all aspects of my life. This path does not make you appear weak or negligent. It shows that you are being realistic and focused.

Remember, your life was probably busy prior to your loved one's health setback. Now you will be adding on all the things that they were responsible for, as well as making decisions for both of you. More than likely, others around you have been in the same situation and are willing to help you sort through those things that are not at the top of your list. Once I followed this simple suggestion, my panic and stress seemed to dissipate. Remember that your main task is to nurture the well-being of the patient as well as yourself. Anything you do to achieve this directive, as simple as it seems, will make your role as a Caregiver meaningful, comforting, and positive.

HOW CAREGIVING AFFECTS YOU:
The Warning Signs

- Sleep deprivation
- Feeling ineffective
- Feeling overwhelmed
- Poor eating habits
- Failure to exercise
- Failure to stay in bed when ill
- Seclusion

- Postponement of or failure to make medical appointments for yourself
- Depression
- Excessive use of drugs or alcohol
- Disorganization
- Misconception of being in control...of everything
- Excess fear, anxiety or worry
- Financial stress
- Unrealistic expectations
- Lack of knowledge or resources
- Lack of effective time management
- Dreading the future
- Job compromises or lack thereof
- Loneliness or sense of avoidance
- Headaches, exhaustion, lack of patience
- Stressed out all the time
- Failure to reach out to others
- Failure to do basic self care
- Forgetting appointments and routine tasks
- Feeling resentful
- Feeling guilty

*When your needs
are taken care of,
the person you care for
will benefit too.*

Take Care of the Caregiver

The one thing that you hear the most as you step into the role of Caregiver is:
Remember to Take Care of Yourself

This statement often becomes generic and undefined. Quite often when you hear someone tell you to take care of yourself, your initial thoughts are:

- What does that even mean to take care of myself?!?
- How can I possibly think about taking care of myself right now?!?
- What happens to the patient while I am doing things for myself?!?
- How will anything get done when I am already overwhelmed?!?
- Have I told you about how nothing went well when I tried to do something for myself?!?

What you need to know, remind yourself of, think about, trust and experience, and remind yourself of again, is:

**When your needs
are taken care of,
the person you care for
will benefit too.**

Grant Me the Serenity
To Accept the Things I Cannot Change;
Courage to Change the Things I Can;
And the Wisdom to Know the Difference.

Self-Care for the Caregiver

After interviewing several patients who noticed significant burnout in their Caregiver, the patients disclosed that they started masking or downplaying their own problems so as not to add to their Caregiver's workload. Unless the Caregiver becomes aware of this occurrence, the outcome can be quite devastating for all parties involved.

Most of us have heard the scenario that if you are involved in an airplane disaster, the first rule is to put on your own oxygen mask before you assist anyone else. A Caregiver told about a time that she was getting on a plane with her elderly mother and this 'rule' came to mind. She convinced herself that her first and foremost task was to take care of her mother's needs before her own. She was asked to try and play out a scene where if something were to happen where she passed out or was injured, then who was going to take care of her mother since she would not be able to? It at least made an impact in her ability to think outside of the Caregiver's box.

Taking care of yourself does not have to be complicated, glamorous, off premises, or costly. If, however, you have someone you trust, who is kind enough to help you every now and then, please consider doing something wonderful for yourself and then try it occasionally. If you do not have a strong support team, then your choices for taking care of yourself become very basic but mandatory. Start slowly trying new things. Always be observant by labeling what you choose, however simple it may seem, as something that is contributing to your taking care of yourself and nurturing your well-being. Your journey will be richer by it, you will be a better Caregiver, and those that surround you and care about you, including the patient, will be relieved. From my conversations with other Caregivers as well as from my own experiences, taking care of yourself is often downplayed or labeled as being self-centered. We all agree, however, that the realization of the importance of self-care is at the forefront when the Caregiver becomes sick or injured and cannot tend to their loved one's needs. Those of us that have unfortunately had this happen, urge you to try and use our experience as a valuable tool in your box of Caregiver's tips!

Caregiver Action Network is a very thorough and informative Facebook page that I read every day. They post articles and various studies that recognize and apply to all areas of Caregiving. It is the most comprehensive and helpful site that I have found so far.

Make a list of things that make you happy.

Make a list of things you do every day.

Compare the Lists.

Adjust Accordingly.

Identifying Personal Barriers

Whenever you get to a point in your caregiving role where you or someone else notices that you are not taking care of yourself, ask yourself:

- What good will I be to the person I care for if I become ill?
- What is the plan for the patient if I cannot take care of them?
- Is not taking care of myself a lifelong pattern?
- What messages do I give myself that get in the way?
- Is this voluntary or did I not have a choice?
- What is my relationship with the patient?
- What is my coping ability?
- What is my awareness of the type, length and details of the illness or injury?
- Am I worried about not wanting to burden others with my situation?

You can read and re-read, hear and hear again, that you need to take care of the Caregiver. Most of the time you get through your day and face the next day with the same determination of taking care of everything—except yourself. You do what you need to do. Perhaps you feel frustrated, exhausted, and sometimes hopeless—but you keep going. The question "What if?" looms two steps behind you and happens when you do not think it will, with no warning and no plan in place. The question "Now What?" is a question you must have answers for, at least as part of a Plan B. If the day comes when you wake up ill and are debilitated for the day and you have no Plan B in place, panic sets in when you cannot even manage to assist your loved one with taking their pills or having a meal. It is not to say that you will not get sick even if you take good care of yourself. You do, however, need to be aware that you must be at your best with self-care, and always have that Plan B in place.

You Can't Pour From An Empty Cup
Take Care of Yourself First

Tips for Self-Care

- Use Positive Statements that identify simple accomplishments: "I am good at sorting my loved one's meds" or "I can exercise 15 minutes today".
- Recognize warning signs (irritability, sleep problems, forgetfulness).
- Identify some sources of stress (too much to do, inability to say no).
- Remember: we can only change ourselves.
- Take time for simple activities (water flowers, read a great book, have a friend over, meditate, pray, take a bubble bath).
- Keep a Journal of things you are grateful for.
- Seek solutions: Identify a problem, list solutions, get opinions.
- Make appointments for personal physical checkups.
- Take special "me" time at least once a day or once a week.
- Communicate constructively: Use "I" messages, be clear, specific, and listen.
- Exercise: Short walks are a great start, or try Yoga or Tai Chi.
- Work on a fun craft (color, bake, create a vision board).

- Maintain good grooming.
- Call someone especially someone who told you to reach out.
- Check for local support groups related to your situation.
- ASK FOR HELP!

Plan B.
Always a Plan B.
Just in Case.

CHAPTER ONE

Do I Bring the Red Shoes

I always like to have a Plan B. Most successful people have a Plan B. The surgeons at the hospital said they always have a Plan B. My quest was figuring out whether bringing my red shoes fit into my Plan A or my Plan B.

Once we had a date set for the transplant surgery, I figured we had plenty of time to prepare for our two-weeks stay. About three months prior to our planned day, I received a phone call from the hospital. They asked how soon we could be there as they had a possible cadaver liver donor for my husband. Mind racing and nerves churning, I arrived promptly to pick up my husband for our long trip to the hospital. Thanks to my amazing friend, we had two suitcases packed containing a change of clothes, pajamas, toothbrushes, a book, and even a candy bar. I must admit that I kept wondering if she had included my red shoes. My passion for shoes seemed to outweigh our focus on the essentials. This experience set the stage for getting serious about my Plan A and Plan B approach.

Each of our many trips to the hospital were different. Occasionally we would have time to pack like we were going on a well-planned vacation, yet other times we arrived with only our cell phones and the clothes on our back. Certainly, there had to be a balance. I have since created a packing list that works for me. The list "What to Bring/Do" is posted at home, included in my cell phone, and written in my journal. I hope this list brings your awareness to the forefront and inspires you to create your own list and always have it handy.

We still have occasions when it is midnight and we are contemplating a trip to the Emergency Room, not knowing if we will be staying overnight or staying for a week. My checklist helps. I have a bag with some items ready to go. I also have an empty bag ready to fill. A side note here is that a backpack is a great go-to bag in case you need to push a wheel chair or for when you have your arms full of your belongings. My packing list eliminates time, stress and worry.

Some of the items from your list can be kept in the trunk of your car ahead of time such as blankets and pillows. Keep in mind that extreme weather can affect the condition of certain items such as makeup or toiletries. The items you forget or cannot bring will now be on a checklist for when you find a place to purchase them, or you can have someone bring them from home.

Just for the record, when I did have the extra time to pack, I always brought the red shoes!

Please make the *What to Bring/Do* list your own, adding items as you think of them. When you have time, prioritize this list into categories. Use a highlighter for the items that you must grab if you only have 5 minutes or less. In my own experiences, my urgent list included: Cell Phone, Charger, Wallet, Water Bottle and a Sweater or Blanket. It is hard to believe, but everything else can be obtained later. It is helpful to always carry around an updated list of medications, and have one posted at home.

The second part of your list is for when you can plan your trip or have more than five minutes. It is wise to have a bag packed with as much of these items as you can, most often possible by purchasing duplicates. I found it helpful to have a bag designated to my clean-up time. It included all my bathroom supplies as well as room for my basic change of clothes. It also contained a waterproof bag for soiled clothes or wet rags/towels. You can launder these items when you arrive at your hotel or pass them on to a person from your "I need help" list. If weather inhibits you from keeping items in the car and you feel you may not get a chance to go home to retrieve your packed bag, then at least keep items like travel blankets, pillows, change of clothes or shoes, extra jacket, and a tote bag. Remember to leave a house key with a neighbor or family member. Again, you can obtain anything you forget, somewhere, somehow. Most importantly, remember to bring your copy of *The Caregiver's Guidebook*.

What to Bring/Do

- Cell phone, charger
- Wallet, credit cards, cash
- List of patient's medications: name/strength/ frequency
- Sweater or sweatshirt

- Blankets (for yourself and a favorite for the patient!)
- Snacks and water bottle
- One or two pillows
- Journal and calendar
- Extra shoes
- Medications and pain relievers for yourself
- Outerwear for daily commutes including umbrella
- Bathroom supplies (listing items separately is recommended!)
- Rag/small towel/wet wipes
- Change of clothes, undergarments for both of you
- Robe, slippers, pajama bottoms for the patient
- A small mirror for the patient's use
- Books/magazines
- Music on phone with earbuds for you and the patient
- Nightlight/flashlight
- Change for vending machine and laundry
- List of contacts (unless you know they are in your phone)
- Home lights on, or on a timer
- Extra key for neighbor

- List of tasks for neighbor to handle while you are gone
- List of bills to pay
- Gas tank full
- Doctors names and numbers
- Quick activated (instant) heat or cold packs
- Box of paperwork or magazines to sort as time allows
- *The Caregiver's Guidebook*!
- Red Shoes

NOTES:

Doctors Diagnose.
Nurses Heal.

Caregivers Make Sense Of It All.

CHAPTER TWO

Can You See Me

Caregivers are Invisible. It is getting better as we create a voice and our needs and concerns move to the forefront. In most hospital settings, especially in any special care unit, the focus is on the patient, and rightfully so. The attention to the Caregiver, however, is crucial because the Caregiver is the middleman that has most of the information available and documented, makes most of the decisions, and is often the key component in the outcome of the patient's care. This invisible status may also be apparent during physician office visits.

My opinions and experiences have resulted in me becoming more assertive yet still polite and respectful of the process. The Caregiver is there to document everything and to be an advocate for the patient's wellbeing. Even though the physicians most often converse directly with the patient, the Caregiver must find a way to document and clarify information about the patient's care and plan of action. Use your journal as a place to document information as it is presented and write down your questions and keep them concise. Most importantly, make sure you understand the information and answers you are given, or ask again.

Doctors: Do not hesitate to ask them to explain something, repeat, or spell anything that you do not understand. The doctor usually gives you a synopsis of the situation then will ask if you have any questions. (My husband's only question was to ask if he could have a room with a view!) The Caregiver must write down any questions or concerns as you will sometimes come up with them later or when you step out for that cup of coffee and miss the doctor's visit. You can always tell your nurse that you have a question for the doctor. Nurses are a great resource. They will connect you to the right person if they cannot help.

Nurses: Your nurse is the key player in your health care experience. They are dedicated to getting to know the patient and their family and taking care of every need, especially in a special care unit. They interact with the doctors, the pharmacy, transport, housekeeping, social workers and anyone else involved in patient care. As Caregiver, you can be of great help to the nurse and learn procedures that you will be responsible for when you get home. Trust, respect, and interaction will make for the best relationship and best care for the patient. On a standard unit in most hospitals, the nurse is taking care of several patients. It may appear that they are not focusing on your patient, however, it may be that they are splitting their time in a way that they have determined to be the best for everyone involved. If you feel frustrated or you have an issue that needs to be addressed in a timelier manner, try to reach out to the Charge Nurse on your unit. If the situation seems complicated or confusing, the Nursing Supervisor will then be able to assist in resolving any concerns.

Pharmacists: The Pharmacy staff in the hospital works closely with the doctors and nurses and are the source for any medication questions and concerns. Be aware that hospitals have guidelines that will affect the patient's use of medications you brought from home. Once you get home, you can ask your local pharmacists any questions that you have regarding the medications or any side effects.

Supplies: Some of the larger hospitals have facilities within the building where you can purchase medical supplies. If not, you can research medical supply locations or not-for-profit organizations that may also have some supplies or equipment that you can borrow or rent. Sometimes nurses can provide you with a sample of what you need that will best suit the patient's home care. Hospital gift shops often have items that will temporarily help get you through your stay.

Social Worker: This person is most likely a key player in your entire experience. They can help you or connect you with someone who can help with inquiries such as: where to park or stay, financial assistance, insurance clarification, or psychological care. This is someone you need to get connected to at the onset of your stay. Whenever you do not know who to ask, contact your social worker.

Psychologist: Most of the larger hospitals have one on staff that either the patient or the Caregiver can utilize. At times their services are not made known, but you can inquire about them.

Patient Advocate: This is someone that is good to know about if you are experiencing some confusing or complicated unresolved issues.

Chaplain: These folks are always available for you or the patient to talk with as your need arises.

NOTE: The glossary at the end of this guidebook will help clarify additional hospital staff members and their basic responsibilities as well as terms that are commonly used in a hospital setting.

Some things that you need to know while staying at the hospital:

- **Where to Clean Up/Freshen Up:** Ask your nurse for suggestions. Have an added carry-along bag of essential items: a small towel, wet wipes, zip lock bags and several travel size necessities. Make and refer to your "What to Bring" list. Sometimes you can use the patient's facilities, however this is not recommended for sanitary reasons. During a patient's ICU stay, if you choose not to leave the hospital, find a restroom that you can use for freshening up. Early morning or late-night hours are the best times to provide you with more privacy in a public setting. Some locations may have showers, so make sure you have items in your carry-along bag that support any option. Having warm water to wash your face or your feet makes for a better start to your day or a more relaxing evening. Your nurse or a staff member can guide you. If you come unprepared, there are usually great travel size supplies available in the hospital gift shop. Bring zip locks and larger bags to store wet items or items for laundry.

- **Where to Sleep:** Except for ICU, there are usually pull-out chairs or couches in the patient's room. It is extremely helpful to have one or two pillows and a couple of warm blankets. Although these may be available from the nurse, quite often they are in short supply. While your loved one is in ICU and you choose not to leave the hospital, you are required to find somewhere in the hospital to spend the night. This usually entails finding a couch, if you are lucky, or two chairs that you can put together. Make sure the area you find is secure, have pillows and warm blankets, and determine a system to secure your belongings. Have a bag for snacks and water and know where the restroom is relative to where you choose to stay. Have a clock or watch, let the nurse know where you are and your phone number, and keep your cell phone on. Know ahead of time what is open for that late-night snack or cup of coffee. Hopefully in the future, more hospitals will start incorporating a better space for the Caregivers.

- **Where to Park:** Most of the large city parking hospital garages have reduced parking rates for their guests. Most of the hospitals can provide you with suggestions of remote parking lots with reduced rates for your long-term stay. Check with your social worker and see if you can locate an offsite indoor parking garage with security that offers reduced weekly rates to hospital patients. I found a safe and secure parking garage a few blocks away that provided reduced costs if you have a patient in the hospital. It cost me the same amount to park for 7 days as it did to park at the hospital for 3 days. It is helpful to take pictures of the lot and the surrounding area and to make notes of cross streets and directions in order to make your trip to the vehicle a simpler task. Sometimes members of the hospital staff also have information on parking places that are nearby.

- **Finding a Hotel:** Most hospitals will give you a list or an 800 number for hotels that offer reduced rates for hospital patients. Some hotels require that your stay be arranged by the social worker. The social worker can also assist you if you have financial restrictions. In certain situations, the hospital puts the patient and Caregiver in a local hotel that will provide transportation back and forth for follow up labs or tests. If the patient is re-hospitalized during this time, the Caregiver must relocate to another room or even another hotel until the patient is once again released. This is great information as it requires additional planning and coordination.

- **Doing Laundry:** Most of the hotels have laundry service, and some have self-serve laundry areas. Make sure you inquire about the details of hours, how many machines, and the cost and the security of the location. A roll of quarters for doing your laundry is a great item to add to your "What to Bring" list.

- **Getting Groceries:** Some of the hotels have kitchen facilities right in your room. This is when you need to research where to buy groceries. Usually you will have more than one grocery store to choose from. If you need to walk any distance and feel like you will be purchasing heavy items, bring an empty pull-behind suitcase with you. You can fit all your groceries in the suitcase and easily pull it back to the hotel.

- **Patient Care:** The nurse will take great care of your loved one. If you are not in a special care unit, there may be periods of time when the nurse or nurse's aide are not readily available to help with basic comfort needs. This is when you can work with your nurse to find out what you can do and where you can obtain the things you need for your loved one. Examples of this might be water, straws, wash rags and towels, toothbrush, new slip resistant socks, extra pillow, portable urinal, etc. Be sure and discuss with your nurse what restrictions the patient has. There will be times when they cannot have water, or cleanup is restricted due to wound care or an upcoming test or procedure. The more you communicate with your nurse, the better off your whole experience will be. Be sure and communicate with your loved one! Ask how they are doing and what they need that day. Help make sure they get their rest and take their walks if it is listed on their activity board. Hold their hand or rub/wash their feet, read them the newspaper or a book, and bring something from home that means a lot to them. Keep things simple, quiet, and honest. Do not assume that you know what they want or what they are thinking. The open communication before coming to the hospital and during their stay will help with their comfort level and the healing process. If you are unsure of what to say or how to handle any part of your stay, be sure and reach out to a professional, whether it is your nurse, the doctor, or even the chaplain or social worker.

- **Guests:** In Special Care Units, quite often there are limitations to the number of guests in a room, as well as restricted visiting times. Do not feel bad informing guests that you have limits on visiting time, both for the patient and yourself. If you have a hard time with this, let your nurse know and she can post a sign or set restrictions for your guests. Remember that the time in the hospital is for recovery, and rest is a big component for success. It is important to remind guests and the staff to wear face masks and wash their hands, especially if they appear to be sick. This concept is good to practice once you get home. Ask your loved one if they are open to having guests. If they want visitors, be sure and create an awareness of their energy level and again do not hesitate to cut short any extensive visits.

- **General Information:** It is imperative throughout your time at the hospital that you know, remember, and keep in mind that the hospital staff and everyone taking care of your loved one is invested in doing their best to take care of their patient. Every now and then situations occur that create doubt, especially when human error creeps into the picture. Your objective as the Caregiver needs to be one of staying calm and patient as you investigate the situation, but more importantly to work with the staff in order to figure out the best solution or find out who will oversee things. Keep yourself updated on how things are progressing with that specific situation, keep accurate and detailed notes, and know who you can go to if you feel as though the process is not moving forward or you are confused with the information presented. The Glossary at the end of this Guidebook will help give you ideas of who might be the next best person to talk to if this rare but possible situation occurs. The staff and the hospital have every intention of providing your loved one with the best care, including plans for moving forward to take the next step in the process. Remember that a simple "thank you for what you do" goes a long way.

NOTES:

*Although it sounds counter-intuitive,
journaling is a social activity.*

CHAPTER THREE

Dear Diary

It is imperative that you purchase a journal, or two, and that it is a size that is easy to carry with you always. This will become your best friend and life-saver. (I have also included blank pages at the end of this book for notes, pictures, etc.) Here are some of the things for which I used my journal:

Medical Contacts: Record each person's name and direct line and an alternative person to contact. Make sure you write down information from *everyone* you meet. You may not realize the significance of this practice until later. Have a pocket section or envelope attached where you can keep business cards.

Maps: (refer to Chapter Four "Am I Going Up or Down") This is a great place to draw your own reference maps. If you must walk the unfamiliar big city streets to go to the parking garage, the grocery store, or the hotel, hand draw a map of each location then list the streets and cross streets to get there. After walking a block, you can take a quick look to make sure you are heading in the right direction. It also helps with planning a route to a new place or series of stops. If you are familiar with the GPS app on your phone, enter the address for where you are heading, then choose the walking icon to take you to your destination.

Daily or Hourly Entries: It is Interesting and helpful to record blood pressure readings, significant health discoveries, procedures and progress, or even an emotional situation. Use this to relay accurate information to the staff, formulate questions for the physicians, and use as a reference down the road.

Vitals and Medications: You will probably be the go-to person for this information and quite often it changes frequently. It is invaluable having this information readily available. Make your own list or use the one in the *List* section at the back of this Guidebook. Use this information as a double-check each time the nurse brings medications to the patient. This will keep you familiar with each medication and provide a double check if there are changes. If you notice something different or new, do not hesitate to ask for clarification, the reason, or any side effects to watch for. It is important that you put a date on this form, so you and the staff know for sure when it has been updated. It is advised that you always make copies of the patient's updated medication list. It becomes easier, safer, and more efficient to have a copy to hand over rather than trying to relay it verbally. When you are in the hospital and give a copy to the nurse, she will use it to update the patient's chart. A pharmacist or doctor may ask for the medication list to review it and check it against what is in the computer. This is a great time to have that extra copy.

Medications

Drug Name	Strength	Quantity	Frequency

People to Thank: This is a big help as each person that lends a hand in any way big or small, receives a place on the list. Go to the gift shop or local store and purchase thank you notes. When you have a few minutes, write a message in a card. You can also hand these off to someone who offers to help you and have them mail them for you. This process is successful since everyone will receive a thank you note, and you will not have to spend time thinking about who did something to help you or gave you a gift, or worse, worrying about who you left out!

Caring Bridge **Posts:** This is a great site to let everyone know updates with one entry rather than calling, texting or emailing several people over and over. Your journal becomes a reference point for composing your *Caring Bridge* posts instead of trying to remember what happened an hour ago or earlier that day. Your guests can use the *Caring Bridge* site to obtain current information on any visiting restrictions or updates on what you or the patient need. I wrote my *Caring Bridge* entries late at night or when I needed to vent my feelings. I saved whatever I wrote to a draft. When I woke up in the morning, more rested, I rewrote my entry trying to keep it positive or humorous, so I would not create worry in all the folks reading it.

Other Lists: There are several other lists that may come to mind that will be helpful for you as you move through this new journey. Start with a blank page at the back of this

Guidebook and write that idea at the top. As you get a thought about the experience that feels unfamiliar or challenging, make a note of how you can make that situation easier or more efficient. Whether you use one of the lists in this Guidebook that is already created for you, or you start one of your own on a blank page, it will help you keep track of things, instead of trying to keep it in your head when you are tired or stressed. The lists that are already created for you can be constantly updated as your experiences expand, and things change. Do not hesitate to purchase another journal if more space is needed, however, it is highly recommended to limit the places where you make notes or keep lists. It is very common for Caregivers to become overwhelmed and unorganized as time goes on. Remember to make your lists work for YOU!

Additional List Ideas:

- Food or other Items to buy
- Things to do (Today/This Week/When You Get Home)
- Appointments to make
- Questions to ask
- Important contacts
- Finances (Budgeting/Prioritizing)
- People to thank
- Patient's Vitals (Blood Pressure/Temperature)

NOTES:

I'm CONFUSED.
no wait…
maybe I'm not.

CHAPTER FOUR

Am I Going Up or Down

As a new Caregiver, sleep was not on the top of my "Things to Do" list. I am sure that in most hospital stays, especially in a critical care unit, sleep for the Caregiver is virtually nonexistent. While standing at the elevator one morning consumed with my warped thinking that I was in total control of everything including my self-care, I encountered the reality that I was sleep deprived when the person standing next to me asked if I was taking the elevator up or down. I realized that I had no idea and could not formulate one, although I knew full well that my intent was to get to the 2nd floor. It was at this point that I knew I needed some tools to help me get by.

Every hospital has a map of their facilities, usually posted on a wall somewhere and/or they have a printed version. When you find one, take a snapshot of it so you have it with you always. You can make notes on the map and put pointers in your journal. When you have time, you can review the map, so you become familiar with the layout and where things are relative to each other. Have your notebook ready when you ask someone in the hospital for directions. Often, they will give you verbal directions that seem to make sense when you hear them, but once you are on your way, you forget the complicated details. Write down what they tell you and read it back to them. Ask if someone can show you the way. You can make notes of landmarks as you travel around. Often, the hospital will not have things marked on the map such as restaurants or shopping, so you will need to inquire about these places and add them to your list. I remember asking if there was a place to send a fax and eventually found it on my own when I had time to wander. I ended up knowing the layout of the hospital like the back of my hand.

The parking garage is another area of confusion, especially in big city hospitals. It seems simple as you pull in and find that one spot to park. You get on the parking garage elevator and make your way to the inside of the hospital, never giving thought to your way out. There are times that you bring your loved one directly to the Emergency Department. Once they are assigned to a room in the hospital, you go along to get settled. This room may be at the opposite end of the hospital from where you originally parked. All the doors, all the floors, and all the spaces merge into one, and you now have no clue where you were or where you are going. Some hospitals have more than one parking garage. Most places have a security car that can drive you around as you attempt to find your car among the thousands of others that are there. In the meantime, you have a patient waiting for you, or you need to move your car, or you are ready to take the patient home. A key solution is your phone. Take pictures of anything you think may be relevant in finding your car and finding your way in and out. Pay attention, look at landmarks, ask questions. The process of taking pictures and making notes is critical while venturing outside of the hospital, especially when you're stressed or tired.

Be Strong Enough
To Stand Alone,

Smart Enough To
Know When You
Need Help,

And Brave Enough
To Ask For It.

CHAPTER FIVE

Complete the Circle

*The second thing we hear the most
as a Caregiver is:*
What Can I Do to Help?

One of the hardest things we must do as a Caregiver is to ask for help. I see it repeatedly when help is offered to someone and they shrug it off with the notion that they will not need it, they do not want to bother anyone, they do not know what they need help with, or even that they do not deserve it. It is imperative that we understand that being on the receiving end is what completes the circle that was intended for us to accept the goodwill of others. Giving and Receiving are equal components of the circle, although most of us are only familiar with or comfortable with the Giving half. We all know it is easy and rewarding to be able to provide help to another human being in need. We all have probably experienced the uncomfortable feeling when it is our turn to receive a gift of help from someone. We need to allow the receiving part of the circle to take place for someone else to experience the glory of giving. I believe we need to practice receiving. Just saying "thank you" is often enough to complete the circle. My husband had to deal with this on a huge scale when he often wondered, "how can I say thank you to someone that donated a portion of their liver to save my life?" His commitment to his donor was that he would take good care of himself and share their story. When the medical world and all its components became bigger than me, I had to reach out and ask for help. Due to an unexpected length of stay in the hospital, our funds became depleted. The thought of asking for money was unimaginable. I forced myself to set up a *Go Fund Me* site and tell my story. To this day, I remember every person (even some I never met before) who contributed to help bring our lives back on track. My commitment to each one of them was, and still is, that I would use the money wisely, then pay it forward whenever I could. It is how I live my life as I am grateful for the chance to know and feel what it is like to complete the circle. It is, I believe, the true gift of Life.

A List to Ask for Help

Creating a list that identifies all the areas with which you need help will benefit you and the people that want to help you. Below is a sample of some things that you can put on your list.

You will get asked many times by many people how they can help. Start with identifying all the things that you do every day and every week, even those things that you may consider irrelevant or mundane. Make a list of the patient's needs and communicate with them about their comfort level and desires. This will help create your checklist that you can hand people when they ask what they can do to help. They can then determine what things they are good at, like to do, or have time to fit in their schedule. Let them decide what or when. Then.... Let Go. Trust the system and each other as you work your list.

Asking for money or gift cards is probably the most difficult, yet the most helpful in moving forward. When someone asks what they can do to help, do not hesitate to suggest gift cards for food or transportation and hand them your personalized list of ideas.

Meals are, most often, the gift of choice. We know the Caregiver and the Patient need to eat and most likely the Caregiver is exhausted. Have a sign-up sheet for meals. There are several great websites that can manage this. Let people know your nutritional restrictions. Prepackaged complete meals in throw away containers is a blessing! When you are home, you can set up a box and/or cooler on your porch where people can place drop-offs in case you are resting or caring for the patient and cannot get to the door.

It is important for you or your representative to reach out to local organizations that can provide you with information and referrals. There are organizations that can help with food, medical supplies, financial assistance, home care, rides, and more. When possible, attend local health fairs to maintain a file of business cards and brochures of services that can help you or someone you know. I have my own list that I am always willing to share. A social worker, home health agency, hospice, physicians, and friends can assist in helping you address your needs. Some of the hospitals have not-for-profit organizations they can refer you to. Support groups are a huge help and can be found online and are often located in your area. Support groups can be for a specific illness or for Caregiving in general. *Caregiver Action Network* is a thorough and informative Facebook page that provides articles or studies that address all components of Caregiving.

You can customize the list below to best suit your life and your new journey. You can even jot down some things as you think of them, then make copies of the list either on your phone so you can forward it or print extra copies that you can hand to someone. You can mention to people that you have a list and that you are open to any ideas they have, since they may know you well enough to figure out what is lacking in your new all-consuming journey.

You may want to customize your list for items you need while you are at the hospital and those items that can wait until you get home. You want to make sure that you do not accumulate too much while you are at the hospital as you will need to pack, carry with, and carry home all your belongings, as well as transporting the patient and any new equipment and medical supplies

Perhaps a sign on your entry door or a message on your voicemail will help clarify your restrictions to all the wonderful folks that want to help you out. This will also help you when the opposite is true and you want visitors, as some people are hesitant to bother you and it might seem that they have forgotten.

Things You Can Help Me With Today

(*Try to indicate days or times that coordinate with your schedule*)

MEALS...
- Set up an online meal signup site
- Consider meals for the caregiver/family
- Define meal needs/restrictions for the patient
- Gift cards for grocery stores or drive through restaurants
- Set up an online grocery delivery service
- Request water bottles, Gatorade, protein drinks, coffee
- Take the Caregiver out for a quick meal
- Determine time and frequency of delivered meals, or assign someone to monitor this

FINANCIAL HELP...

- Cash
- Gift cards for cash, food, medical supplies, travel
- Organize my bills
- Set up a budget
- Organize and set up tax forms

IN THE HOSPITAL...

- Bring or purchase a meal
- Give a packet of notecards
- Provide a book of stamps
- Give a coin purse of quarters for laundry or vending machines
- Provide a gift card for food or gas
- Purchase or make a keepsake that provides hope
- Bring or purchase a portable phone charger
- Provide a travel coffee mug and/or water bottle
- Bring snacks
- Offer to make phone calls
- Take back excess items home that are no needed
- Bring items from your home (mail or change of clothes)

- Stay with patient to allow Caregiver time away to rest or shop
- Offer to take home or do laundry
- Provide a beautiful, small and lightweight Journal
- Give a beautiful pen
- Provide a lightweight pouch for paperwork and journal

HOUSEKEEPING...
- Dust
- Vacuum
- Shake out rugs
- Wash floors
- Clean bathroom
- Change sheets
- Do laundry
- Empty wastebaskets
- Take out garbage

OUTDOOR MAINTENANCE...
- Mow lawn
- Weed garden
- Water flowers
- Rake leaves or shovel snow
- Sweep

RUN ERRANDS...
- Pick up prescriptions
- Shop for groceries
- Drive to doctor appointments
- Assist in banking transactions

CHILDREN...
- Drive to _____
- Pick up from _____
- Help with homework
- Pack lunches
- Babysit

PET CARE...
- Feed pets
- Walk dog
- Pick up pet food
- Take to vet appointment
- Clean up yard/litter box

MISC...
- Set up medications
- Organize mail
- Organize bills for payment
- Other

Life is Short

Take the Trip
Buy the Shoes
Eat the Cake

CHAPTER SIX

Enjoy Your Life

After four years of appointments, procedures and two major surgeries, the physicians, surgeons, and hospital staff continue to thank us for being so positive. They told us it helps with healing. We trusted and believed in them and we solved any setbacks with humor and a we-can-do-this approach. As his recovery period began, my husband was often fatigued or not feeling well, and follow-up appointments were abundant. Vacations or trip planning, even if they were short or close to home, were out of the question. We decided to stick with one-day adventures such as concerts or art shows or a day in the park. That way if we had to cancel at the last minute, it was not a huge disruption or disappointment. When we look back at our calendar and photographs from the prior years, we realize how much fun we had!

After one of my husband's hospital stays, one of the surgeons came in to say hello. He looked my husband in the eye and said, "go home and enjoy your life." At that moment, we both smiled and agreed with his sincere statement. On the way home, and several days thereafter, we started to question what the doctor said. "Isn't that something you hear when you are old or sick?" and, "Was he trying to tell us something?" After discussing it further, we decided that these are great words to live by. This is something we all need to hear every day! We were already living that way, and now feel assured that no matter what happens tomorrow, that we have really enjoyed our lives today.

Glossary

The following descriptions are meant to give you a basic understanding of positions and procedures related to hospital settings. The descriptions are general or generic and may not apply to the hospital you are associated with, or the title may be different based on the hospital and its affiliates.

Advance Directive
A written statement of a person's wishes regarding medical treatment, often including a living will, made to ensure those wishes are carried out should the person be unable to communicate them to a doctor. A Medical Power of Attorney is a legal document that authorizes someone you trust to make medical decisions on your behalf. If you want to choose one person to speak for you on health care matters, and someone else to make financial decisions, you can do separate financial and health care powers of attorney.

Case Manager

A Registered Nurse who develops, implements, evaluates and coordinates patient care plans. They serve as a liaison between patients, their families, and healthcare providers.

Catheter

A soft hollow tube which is passed into the bladder to drain urine, usually after surgery. These are often necessary for people who cannot empty their bladder in the usual way and are most often temporary.

Certified Nursing Assistant (CNA)

Responsible for assisting patients with all basic personal care activities they might have trouble with on their own, including but not limited to, bathing, dressing, skin and oral care, bedding changes. They are required to bring all patient concerns and issues to their supervisor.

Chain of Command in Hospitals:

Managers ensure that workers complete tasks and activities, are safety compliant, and provide proper patient care. Upper level management establishes a higher level of direction, policies, procedures, and productivity. Generally, in a hospital setting if your needs or questions exceed the response your bedside nurse can provide, you can inquire to speak with the Charge Nurse and/or the Nursing Supervisor.

Chaplain

An ordained clergy member who provides non-denominational psycho-social-spiritual guidance, representing a variety of faiths. They are great listeners that work collectively and collaboratively alongside other health care professionals.

Charge Nurse/Patient Care Leader

Supervises and supports a nursing staff, while also treating a limited number of patients. They are responsible for maintaining a high level of patient care, evaluating other nurses and acting as an educational resource for other nurses. They have the same responsibility as a Nursing Supervisor but are Unit Specific rather than Hospital Wide.

Dietician

An expert in nutrition and the regulation of diet. They alter the patient's nutrition based on each patient's medical condition and individual needs. Dieticians are regulated healthcare professionals licensed to assess, diagnose, and treat nutritional problems by helping the patient set goals and prioritize.

Do Not Resuscitate (DNR)

A medical order written by a doctor, agreed to by the patient, and understood by the family, that instructs health care providers not to revive the patient if their heart stops or they stop breathing.

Fellow

A physician who has completed their residency and elects to complete further training in a specialty. The Fellow is a fully credentialed physician who participates in patient care under the direction of attending physicians in that specialty.

Home Health Care

Supportive care provided in the home. Care may be provided by licensed healthcare professionals who provide medical treatment needs or by professional caregivers who provide daily assistance to ensure the activities of daily living are met.

Hospitalist

Physicians whose primary professional focus is the general medical care of hospitalized patients. Their activities include patient care, teaching, research, and leadership related to Hospital Medicine. They do not see patients in an office-based setting.

Intensive Care Unit (ICU)

A unit that provides specialized treatment given to patients who have an acute illness or injury and require critical medical care. ICU Nurses commonly have only one or two patients rather than five or six in standard hospital rooms.

Interventional Radiology (IR)

A procedure that provides minimally invasive image-guided diagnosis and treatment with less risk and less pain than open surgery.

Intubation

A standard procedure that involves placing a flexible plastic tube through the mouth into a person's airway. Doctors often perform this before surgery or in emergencies to give medicine or help a person breathe.

Medical Records

A chronological record of a patient's health and medical history and is a systematic documentation of care across time within one health care provider's jurisdiction, including but not limited to care and treatments received, test results, diagnoses, and medications taken. Under HIPAA you have access to your health records

MELD Score

Model for End-Stage Liver Disease, or MELD, is a scoring system used to determine the severity of chronic liver disease for transplant planning for patients 12 years and older. Hospitals and the government use the score to prioritize allocation. The value ranges from 6 to 40, using three easily obtained laboratory values. The closer you are to 40 places you in a more critical state of receiving a transplant.

Negative Test Results

A test result that shows the substance or condition the test is supposed to find is NOT present at all or is present but in normal amounts.

Nurse Manager

Responsible for supervising nursing staff, overseeing patient care, making management and budgetary decisions, setting work schedules and coordinating meetings. They have the responsibility of a specific Unit with 24/7 accountability for their employees.

Nurse Practitioner

An advanced practice registered nurse, licensed by the Nursing Board, can assesses patient needs, and can order, interpret, and diagnose lab tests. They can also diagnose illness or disease, prescribe meds, and formulate treatment and plans. Traditionally the focus is based more on a whole person/wellness approach.

Nursing Supervisor
Responsible for managing staff, overseeing patient care, and ensuring adherence to established policies and procedures. They also act as an interface between their staff, their patients, the patients' families, and between their staff and the hospital's physicians.

Palliative Care
Specialized medical care for people with a serious illness, focused on providing relief from the symptoms, pain, and stress of the illness. The goal is to improve quality of life for both the patient and the family.

Physician Assistant
Medical providers who are licensed to diagnose and treat illness and disease and can prescribe medication for patients and manage treatment plans. They often serve as the patient's principal healthcare provider. They may assist doctors in surgical procedures but are not licensed to perform surgery themselves. A Physician Assistant has a master's degree and must

work in conjunction with a doctor. Traditionally the focus is based more on a medical model.

Registered Nurse (RN)/Licensed Practical Nurse (LPN)
RN's primarily administer medication, treatments, and offer educational advice to patients and the public. LPN's usually provide more basic nursing care and are responsible for the comfort of the patient.

Social Worker
Responsible for helping patients and their families navigate life's most challenging moments. In many healthcare teams, Social Workers with an MSW degree, provide mental health assessments and counseling to help cope with problems the patients and their families are/will be facing.

Surrogate Decision Maker
A substitute decision maker (family member, friend, guardian) that makes medical treatment decisions for patients that lack the ability to make and communicate decisions about medical care, and do not have a Power of Attorney for Health Care, a Living Will Declaration, or other advance directives. The decisional capacity is determined by a physician.

Teaching Hospital

A hospital that partners with medical and nursing schools, education and research centers to improve healthcare through training, education, and research.

Trauma Level 1

A hospital that treats trauma patients and are equipped and staffed to provide total care for patients suffering from major traumatic injuries such as falls, motor vehicle accidents, etc. Treatments include prevention and rehab.

Trauma Level 2

A hospital that includes immediate definitive care for all injured patients with 24-hour coverage by general surgeons, orthopedic and neuro surgeons, anesthesiologists, emergency medicine, radiology and critical care.

Lists

The following pages contain the lists that are contained within the chapters of this Guidebook in order to give you easy, quick access.

You can also go to www.caregiversguidebook.com to access these Lists to print for your personal use.

There are several other lists that may come to mind that will be helpful for you as you move through this new journey. Start with a blank page and write that idea at the top. As you get a thought about the experience that feels unfamiliar or challenging, make a note of how you can make that situation easier or more efficient. Whether you use one of the lists in this Guidebook that is already created for you, or you start one of your own on a blank page, it will help you to keep track of things, instead of trying to keep it in your head while you are tired or stressed. The lists that are already created for you can be constantly updated as your experiences expand and things change. Do not hesitate to purchase another journal if more space is needed, however, it is highly recommended to limit the places where you make notes or keep lists. It is very common for Caregivers to become overwhelmed and unorganized as time goes on. Remember to make your lists work for YOU!

Additional List Ideas:
- Food or other items to buy
- Things to do (Today/This Week/When You Get Home)
- Appointments to make
- Questions to ask
- Important contacts
- People to thank
- Finances (Budgeting/Prioritizing)
- Patient's vitals
  (Blood Pressure/Temperature/Pain Level)

MEDICATIONS

(*NOTE: Make Several Copies of This Form*)

Drug Name	Strength	Quantity	Frequency
(Drug name)	(__ mg)	(2)	(Twice a Day)

Medications available to print www.caregiversguidebook. com

CAREGIVING DYNAMICS:
Questions to Consider

- What is your relationship to the patient?
- Will you be the main caregiver?
- Do you live with the patient?
- Do you live nearby?
- Are you organized?
- Are you assertive?
- Do you already take good care of yourself?
- What is your financial status?
- Do you know the financial status of the patient?
- Will you be the only one taking care of this person?
- What does your normal day look like?
- Will you be responsible for taking this person to appointments?
- Does the patient have organized and accessible records?
- Has the patient talked with you about their care?
- Do you have a caregiving plan and do all family members understand and agree with the Plan?
- Have you been in the medical setting before?
- Do you have access to insurance policies (medical and prescription)s?
- Do you have power of attorney?

- Are you set up for impromptu hospital stays?
- Do you need referrals?
- Can you take pictures with your phone?
- Are you going to be able to shop and cook for special meals?
- Do you have good nutrition in place for yourself?
- Do you have a reliable vehicle?
- Do you know how to ask for help?
- Do you know what to ask help for?
- Is the home where the patient is staying clean and safe?
- Are you okay with travel in bad weather?
- Do you have a list of what to bring on hospital stays both planned and impromptu?
- Do you know who to call after hours?
- Do you have contacts set up in your phone (numbers and email)?
- Do you have someone set up to take care of pets, mail, lights?
- Is your place of employment aware of your new lifestyle?
- Do you have a network established: family, friends, health care?
- Do you have an action plan for the next phase?

- Do you have an action plan for the unexpected?
- Did you consider a life alert device and/or medical bracelet?
- Do you have a list of current medications posted in several locations?
- Do you have a notification site set up to disseminate the patient's health status?
- Are you aware of forms that your hospital requires to enable you to make and discuss health decisions for the patient?
- Are you comfortable discussing health changes with the patient?
- Do you have a way to efficiently communicate with others?
- Do you know who to talk to if you cannot answer these questions?
- Do you have a Plan B?

Caregiving Dynamics: Questions to Consider available to print www.caregiversguidebook.com

HOW CAREGIVING AFFECTS YOU:
The Warning Signs

- Sleep deprivation
- Feeling ineffective
- Feeling overwhelmed
- Poor eating habits
- Failure to exercise
- Failure to stay in bed when ill
- Seclusion
- Postponement of or failure to make medical appointments for yourself
- Depression
- Excessive use of drugs or alcohol
- Disorganization
- Misconception of being in control of everything
- Excess fear, anxiety or worry
- Financial stress
- Unrealistic expectations
- Lack of knowledge or resources
- Lack of effective time management
- Dreading the future
- Job Compromises or lack thereof
- Loneliness or sense of avoidance
- Headaches, exhaustion, lack of patience

- Stressed out all the time
- Failure to reach out to others
- Failure to do basic self care
- Forgetting appointments and routine tasks
- Feeling resentful
- Feeling guilty

How Caregiving Affects You: The Warning Signs available to print www.caregiversguidebook.com

TIPS FOR SELF-CARE

- Use positive statements that identify simple accomplishments: "I am good at sorting his meds" or "I can exercise 15 minutes today".
- Recognize warning signs (irritability, sleep problems, forgetfulness).
- Identify some sources of stress (too much to do, inability to say no).
- Remember: we can only change ourselves.
- Take time for simple activities (water flowers, read a great book, have a friend over, meditate, pray, take a bubble bath).
- Keep a Journal of things for which you are grateful.
- Seek solutions: Identify a problem, list solutions, get opinions.
- Make appointments for personal physical checkups.
- Take special "me" time at least once a day or once a week.
- Communicate constructively: Use "I" messages, be clear, specific, and listen.
- Exercise: Short walks are a great start, or try Yoga or Tai Chi.
- Work on a fun craft (color, bake, create a vision board).

- Maintain good grooming.
- Call someone especially someone who told you to reach out.
- ASK FOR HELP!

WHAT TO BRING/DO

- Cell phone, charger
- Wallet, credit cards, cash
- List of patient's medications: name/strength/ frequency
- Sweater or sweatshirt
- Blankets (for yourself and a favorite for the patient!)
- Snacks and Water Bottle
- One or two pillows
- Journal and calendar
- Extra shoes
- Medications and pain relievers for yourself
- Outerwear for daily commutes including umbrella
- Bathroom supplies (listing items separately is recommended!)
- Rag/small towel/wet wipes
- Change of clothes, undergarments for both of you
- Robe, slippers, pajama bottoms for the patient
- A small mirror for the patient's use
- Books/magazines
- Music on phone with earbuds for you and the patient

- Nightlight/flashlight
- Change for vending machine and laundry
- List of contacts (unless you know they are in your phone)
- Home lights on, or on a timer
- Extra key for neighbor
- List of tasks for neighbor to handle while you are gone
- List of bills to pay
- Gas tank full
- Doctors names and numbers
- Quick activated (instant) heat or cold packs
- Box of paperwork or magazines to sort as time allows
- *The Caregiver's Guidebook*!
- Red Shoes

What to Bring/Do available to print www.caregiversguide-book.com

THINGS YOU CAN HELP ME WITH TODAY

(Try to indicate days or times that coordinate with your schedule)

MEALS

- Set up an online meal signup site
- Consider meals for the caregiver/family
- Define meal needs/restrictions for the patient
- Gift cards for grocery stores or drive through restaurants
- Set up an online grocery delivery service
- Request water bottles, Gatorade, protein drinks, coffee
- Take the Caregiver out for a quick meal
- Determine time and frequency of delivered meals, or assign someone to monitor this

FINANCIAL HELP

- Cash
- Gift cards for cash, food, medical supplies, travel
- Organize my bills
- Set up a budget
- Organize and set up Tax Forms

IN THE HOSPITAL

- Bring or purchase a meal
- Give a packet of notecards
- Provide a book of stamps
- Give a coin purse of quarters for laundry or vending machines
- Provide a gift card for food or gas
- Purchase or make a keepsake that provides hope
- Bring or purchase a portable phone charger
- Provide a travel coffee mug and/or water bottle
- Bring snacks
- Offer to make phone calls
- Take back excess items home that are not needed
- Bring items from your home (mail or change of clothes)
- Stay with patient to allow for Caregiver time away to rest or shop
- Offer to take home or do laundry
- Provide a beautiful, small and lightweight Journal
- Give a beautiful pen
- Provide a lightweight pouch for paperwork and journal

HOUSEKEEPING

- Dust
- Vacuum
- Shake out rugs
- Wash floors
- Clean bathroom
- Change sheets
- Do laundry
- Empty wastebaskets
- Take out garbage

OUTDOOR MAINTENANCE

- Mow lawn
- Weed garden
- Water flowers
- Rake leaves or shovel snow
- Sweep

RUN ERRANDS

- Pick up prescriptions
- Shop for groceries
- Drive to doctor appointments
- Assist in banking transactions

CHILDREN
- Drive to _____
- Pick up from _____
- Help with homework
- Pack lunches
- Babysit

PET CARE
- Feed pets
- Walk dog
- Pick up pet food
- nake to vet appointment
- Clean up yard/litter box

MISC
- Set up medications
- Organize mail
- Organize bills for payment
- Other

Things You Can Help Me With Today available to print
www.caregiversguidebook.com

FOOD/ITEMS TO PURCHASE

PATIENT'S VITALS
(Blood Pressure/Temperature/Pain Level)

THINGS TO DO
(Today/This Week/When Arrive Home)

APPOINTMENTS TO MAKE

QUESTIONS TO ASK

IMPORTANT CONTACTS

FINANCES

THANK YOU LIST

Conclusion

At some point in our lives, we all will become a Caregiver. It is quite a journey and more than likely one that you have never had before. It will have happy and sad times rolled into one You are not the only one that has or will go through this and all the rest of us Caregivers are cheering you on! You can do this! You are ready and will learn the ropes. You will learn who to reach out to and when. You will learn to love yourself. You will learn that post traumatic stress is part of the process and it is not a flaw. You will learn that you are human and will make mistakes or bad decisions. You will learn that no matter what happens, as you take care of yourself, stay positive, and reach out to the rest of us that want to help you, that you will be okay. Congratulations from all the Caregivers that have paved the way for your success in your new role. Embrace the title and pave the way for others that will follow.

Take Care of Yourself, Enjoy Your Life, and Bring the Red Shoes

About the Author

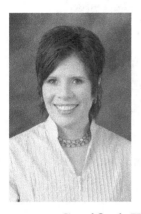

Barbara A. Stewart, Certified Wellness Coach, Certified Pharmacy Technician, Licensed Massage Therapist, and Self-Taught Caregiver believes wellness to be a proactive dedication to health through prevention.

Barbara's workshops and one-on-one sessions provide support, guidance, and healing options, inspired by her positive, humorous, and compassionate approach.

The Caregiver's Guidebook supports Barbara's mission of providing a voice and creating comfort for the caregiver. Her presentation that coincides with this book adds elements of personal animation and interesting stories.

Email: imb2002@att.net
Website: www.caregiversguidebook.com
      www.imb.massagetherapy.com
Facebook: Barb Stewart
Linkedin: Barb Stewart
Twitter: @BarbStewart2002
Instagram: barbstewart1954

Acknowledgments

Thank you to:

My husband, for being a good patient and for showing that humor and a positive attitude really helps with the healing process.

Amy, for the selfless act of being a transplant donor, and for bringing live donor awareness to the forefront.

My friends, clients, and colleagues, for providing unconditional support and encouragement.

The hospital staff, the transplant team, and other supportive services, for their relentless dedication.

Caregivers that I interviewed, for sharing their personal stories, for helping me understand the depth of being a Caregiver, and for their continued example of strength and endurance.

My mother, for being my Caregiver role model, and the person who cheered me on to the finish line throughout my life.

My sister, for providing me a better understanding of the challenges while caring for a loved one with a progressive disease, and **My brother and his wife,** for lovingly taking care of our mother. .

Lyn, for her expertise as our Coach and Healing Touch Practitioner, and for her comfort, help and humor.

Eileen, a professional writer, editor, teacher, and a true friend who nurtured and encouraged my ideas and enthusiasm to help make this guidebook a reality

NOTES

NOTES

NOTES

NOTES

NOTES

NOTES

CPSIA information can be obtained
at www.ICGtesting.com
Printed in the USA
JSHW020454280920
8208JS00003B/100